The Story Of A Sad Woman

I0705614

By: Matilda Reese

"I decided that I was gonna kill myself today...."

-Part 1-

Chapter 1

Carefully touching the eagle fern leaves to watch the leaf curl in. I like this type of fern. I like all plants, but especially ferns. Most people ignore them but they are so cool. There are so many interesting things about ferns that nobody notices. I can feel Ms. Amber, my therapist, staring daggers into me. I keep my finger in the curled-up plant. It feels like a baby's hand around your finger, encapsulating a baby's innocence As a fern is younger it's as sensitive as a baby. It is more receptive to what is happening when it grows older like an adult. "You're getting worse…" Ms. Amber breaks the silence in possibly the worst way. I don't even bother to look over my shoulder, I know how she looks at me. Disappointment.

That's all her face right now I bet. "And you know you are, but you won't do anything to fix it." God, I hated that. She said it all the goddamn time. I told the day I started this stupid therapy session that I wouldn't change. I hated to admit it but I did grow a little, but it didn't last. Nothing I did made anything better besides one thing. Drugs, drinking, sex, gambling, gardening, reading, it never did anything besides painting. I loved paintings. Studying it and practicing.

My favorite artist was Basquiat. His artwork was phenomenal, and I've always wanted that creative artwork. But no matter how I tried to do the same thing with his artwork, I always created a monster.

I feel a monster inside. I know it, and so does Dr. Amber. So, I stick to only learning about art.

"Tell me more about your artwork." She asks me this all the time. I hate it, I know she thinks that this talk will get us a breakthrough, but it won't. I know exactly what's wrong with me, and it's for me to know and for her to never know. It is always the same goddamn line, "I am your therapist."

Well I didn't fucking ask for that, did I. Never did I ever want to have a therapist. "Okay, how have you been this week, your physiatrist called me and said you renewed your anxiety pills again this week." She pulled out a piece of paper from her desk. With how much paperwork she has about me, she should have a whole filing cabinet dedicated to me. The paper she pulled out was a form of a refill prescription. "I am getting more and more from your doctor. What is going on is that you would need these many anxiety pills." I knew I had to lie, if she knew the real reason I had taken so many pills, I would be here for multiple fucking hours. I hated when she did this, it wasn't a therapist appointment it was interrogation now. I wanted to leave. Turning back around to face her, I slightly turn the bowl of chocolate kisses that are there. Walking back over to the desk, it felt like time slowed. I could see Dr. Amber's face of disappointment. She slowly blinked and her eyes watched me sit down. It felt like 30 years before I sat down in the chair. White cushions with walnut for the arms rests and the legs. Fits the bleachy tone of her office. The only thing I didn't like in her office was that she had a dark wood table, while the rest of the wood was walnut. Bad fucking taste. I can't look her in the eyes, I can only look at her hand when they move to write on the damned paper. Yellow legal pads are what she uses when writing.

I stare at her desk again and again. And every time I can tell you exactly the grain that the desk has. I know she keeps writing about how I don't keep eye contact, I answer questions vaguely, and I am overly focused on little details in her office. I know she's writing this because when Dr. Amber led me out of the room, I was glazed and mentally scanned the gross yellow paper. Another glance around the office again, no matter how many times I remember the office there's always another fucking leak on the ceiling. Dr. Amber told me that there was a break room above us, which must have been the spillage. I have never believed her, she's a therapist she can lie so easily. Another reason I don't believe her is because I would hear a lot more footsteps above us if it was a break room.

I look back down at the floor with the same carpet I see every Thursday. 1,202 is how many waves this carpet has. It's a nice navy blue, by itself. With oak it's okay, they are both dark undertones colors, but with walnut it's bad. The walnut has a red undertone instead. 'She's still writing' I think as I stare at her hand, she has nice handwriting. Cursive but not enough to where every letter looks the same. "What about nightmares… any more nightmares?" Knowing I can't lie anymore so I give in this time. "One last night…"

"Okay..tell me about it"

I glance at her, I don't want to. But she'll be pushing to hear. I don't want to tell her.

"It had a moose"

"Hmm…okay, tell me more"

She writes on the yellow legal paper.

"It was winter, and I was looking at them through the window"

"Okay…anything else?'

She looks at me while she writes, I hate that she can do that.

"Um…it was all in black and gray, but darker and more in the blue area."

I didn't want to tell her, but I feel this relief that lifts from my shoulders when I talk about my dreams. I hate and love that fucking feeling.

"Besides that, nothing else"

"Okay, well looking back at some of my other notes…I noticed that the moose and grayscale appear more and more."

God, next she's gonna tell me she looked it up.

"So, I looked up those meanings,"

Fucking called it

"And moose represents being more adaptive and having strength and resilience"

Goddammit

"And a grayscale in dreams is a sense of loss, loneliness, and/ or emotional repression"

Oh, great, more things to talk about next time. How wonderful! Looking down at my shoes, I turn them inwards and then out three times. That's my routine, I look at my shoes and then the time. If I was about 10 seconds it makes me feel better about looking at the time. It's 3:59. 1 more minute.

She's still talking, oh my god.

4:00

Finally…this nightmare is over. As much as I don't like these sessions, I do like the idea of having someone to talk to. Nonetheless whoever I talk to about my problem always finds it to be too much for even them.

Chapter 2

Walking into the apartment, I lived in it for 2 years, and it never felt like home to me. In the green-colored rotting apartment. 3rd floor, 58th apartment, unfortunately, I couldn't get a better-numbered floor or apartment. Something like the 2nd floor in the 25th apartment. I like that.
No matter how ugly and depraved this building may be I still like to keep things tidy. I put my Doc Martens on the shoe rack. They are right next to my vans and nikes. Everything goes from most worn to less worn. Just like my closet. In the middle is the most worn, to the left is the lesser worn long sleeve and to the right is the lesser worn short sleeve. I counted everything before, and I have exactly 122 pieces of clothes in my closet, (including winter gear, hats and gloves, socks and underwear).
I love my Doc Martens but they sometimes get a bit much to wear.
I hear two meows from the hallway of the apartment.
My two babies!
A long gray-haired cat trots over to greet me. It has pricing yellow eyes and a rail that looks like a candy cane when she is happy. Another cat, a domestic shorthair tabby. She is mostly caramel with a few spots of brown mixed in. She has green eyes and a tail that sits low. She had high ears and short whiskers. Finally my all-white domestic Manx cat. She has no tail, and she doesn't meow much, but she is adorable. They all contrast and complement each other. They are the ones that I can truly say that I love. I would go to the end of the world for my cats.
Walking over to the moldy kitchen, I grab my normal lunch. I never really have anything in my pantry. Mostly just pasta, oatmeal, chicken, and fries. When I do feel like I deserve something I'll make ribs, and I've only had those two times since living on my own. I wish I could say that I only have this little food because I don't have money, but that's not it. I make a steady income as a TV assistant for weather and news. It's that I don't eat what I need to.
After a mental breakdown, the company decided to give me paid time off. I hated that decision. I have nothing to do for the time being. I need something to do. This urge that I have in my heart to make perfection is aching.
Knowing that I won't ever agree with the people at work, I eat. Eating is difficult because my brain will not work. What I mean by that is my brain won't swallow or chew. I don't know why it happens but it does. It's hard to eat when you know

that you may forget how to swallow and then collapse and die. The weird thing is this only occurs when I am alone. When I am in a public space I am a normal person eating and drinking. My brain works then. But once I get home, I forget everything.

I remember just how to eat, I remember how to walk or just breathe. I assume it's the apartment, I know that it's depression, but also how many bad things that have happened, it adds up. There is an aura of sadness, around me and this apartment. When together we clash and grow even stronger as a storm cloud. Oatmeal is easy, that's why I have so much of it. I can swallow and not chew, it's easy and I don't have to think I am gonna die. Besides the taste of maple and brown sugar with peanut butter, it's truly delicious! I put my bowl in the sink, the only dish. It's centered, I filled it with water perfectly, not a drop outside. I'll wash it tomorrow, and let the dish soak.

It's routine

I get my cat's food, my body is on autopilot now. The feeling is like my brain is in a stage and my body goes on muscle memory. I like this feeling, it's freeing.

If I had imagined what death felt like, this would be it. It's nice.

I wanted to be dead, well not dead per se. You could say that I wanted to disappear. I wanted to be a dead leaf floating on a calm river. My life was too much, too much noise, lights, stress, and pain. A pearl in a clam shell. There's too much work that goes into dying. Especially the work of suicide, the deciding how you're gonna die. Going through with it and how long it may take, and you also risk being brought back. There's too much work, I just want to disappear. This also makes people less prone to worrying about me, in their minds everyone has wanted to disappear at one point. It's not as worrisome as telling someone you're gonna kill yourself.

Getting out of this train of thought, I am in my bed.

Autopilot.

My bed is a queen size with dark blue sheets and pillowcases. My room has blackout sheets, it is the time I can escape from the real world. With me and my cats, watching some trash TV. Wallowing in my self emptiness and pity.

I like trash TV, it makes me feel even the tiniest bit better about who I am as a person. Hey, I may be a self-hating bitch, but at least I am not spoiled or entitled, I can at least count that as a plus.

What I find funny is how I treat my cats better than myself. They have their monthly checkups, keeping up with shots, while I haven't been to the doctor in 6 years. They get the highest quality food, while everything I get is discounted at Walgreens. I always knew my animals were better than me in every aspect. That's why I have them, they give me a sense of soul, my cats. They're fucking everything to me.

I love them more than myself.

The final destination is on. I loathe this movie. Because it gets to me, physiologically. One time I was extra cautious and didn't go somewhere or do something I missed death. Now this entity is chasing after me, using everything around me to try and kill me. It's my worst nightmare.

My mortality.

That's my worst fear.

Most people think they're aware of mortality but they're not. They don't realize that the smallest things can kill you. They are only aware that they will enviably

die. People don't understand that it can happen at any point, in any capacity. The most mundane things can kill you. Cooking, bathing, showering, sleeping, literally anything. And it's worse when you're aware of it. When you know you can die anywhere, and at any time, you're terrified of everything.
Being aware of your mortality is a nightmare that no one deserves.
No matter how many times I try not to think about it, the worries always come back. They can never leave my head. Everything I look at can be a death trap, stairs, car, chairs, AC, TV, or any fucking thing that can kill me.
Mortality is the bane of everything's existence.

Chapter 3

Even though I got paid leave, I made sure that I had some work. If I didn't I was sure I was gonna go insane. My job from my leave was to look over the script for the hosts. I did theater, backstage theater. Helping the actual starring kids, I had this need to be in the shadows. The roar of the crowd frightened me, if I heard the crowd while I was on stage I would probably start crying hysterically. I like having to know things, and how they work.
The only thing I would change was how much Cathline talked. I fucking hate Cathline, I know she's cheating on her husband. While on top of that, she was too fucking loud. She needed to shut the fuck up. I would erase some of the lines, extra that were put in to make it seem more friendly. I hated that part of the morning TV, we watch the TV for news from people we don't know. I am not friendly with those people, I watch the fucking news for the stuff I don't know about, not act like I am talking about this self with friends.
Every time I heard Cathline my fist would clench, breaking skin with my nails. Her voice was scratching, like someone who just recovered from a cold. I don't hate many things.
But I do hate Cathline.
Getting done with work was quick, I tried my hardest to at least leave bed for it, but in the end, I stayed. My bed was my safe place, where I felt pleasure, sadness, anger, and fear.
I liked my life a certain way, I've always had. I wanted to graduate from a state college, get a good-paying corporate job, get married, have 3 kids, and a dog, know my husband is cheating but not say anything and die. That's what I wanted. A simple life, a quiet life. Where there would be enough people at my funeral for people to think, "This is a lot more people than I thought would show up". Not too much of a notable person, but just enough that some people would care. I liked those 90's dream families you would see on TV, that's what I wanted. I wanted that simple life. Except I am not, I don't have that simple life. I live in a crappy apartment with 3 cats. It turns out I am infertile, have no significant other, and have a TV technician job.
My life is fucking shit.
But at least whenever I look at my cats, I can feel somewhat happy.

It hurt a lot when I found out I was infertile. At the time I was rounding to my late 20s and I had a house with a 4 year relation with my boyfriend. We knew that we were in a good place to have kids. We tried and tried for at least 5 months before I went to the doctor. That's when we got the news of my infertility. It was April 2016 when we went to the doctor. My boyfriend at the time was reassuring me that everything was fine with me. He was in denial that it might have been him that was the problem. Even though that was an option in my head, I had a feeling that I knew what the doctor was gonna say. When we got the news it was 1:26 pm, my boyfriend had been quiet the entire time, and when we got out of the office he just started screaming. It was a kick in the gut already from my infertility and now he was screaming how horrible this was. It was all too much, I ended up throwing up on the dashboard, at least that shut him up. When we got home, we ordered a supreme pizza, with no mushrooms. As we ate, he brought up the words.
"I think we should break up"
When I countered with adoption, he said that he wanted the kid to be his, biologically that is. Depression hit in those 30 minutes so hard that I agreed. We sold the house and I moved to Washington State.
This was the single nerve that would cause the fern to curl in.
My dad got diagnosed with cancer, and the strong man I once knew was rooting away in a nursing home. It was too much. My employer sat me down and told me that I had to go to a therapist and get some help, otherwise I would be let go. At least my therapy was covered by my insurance.
My life was a graph chart, going up, going down, and having its middle points. This was a middle point.
My life was okay, but I knew I could live with this being my entire life. Even for me, this was depressing, I mean, shit, my cats have more food and furniture than me! What kind of fucking life is this!

That day I knew I was going to kill myself.

Chapter 4

On my calendar, June 8th, 2019 was circled in red, labeled with death day. It is currently May 18th, 2019, 3 weeks is what I have left.
Perfect
I knew that this would be more planning, and I was prepared. I have around 3,0000 dollars saved, so I can still end up paying rent and getting the bare minimum of groceries. Another thing I had to worry about was the therapy sessions. This is one point I was happy that I did theater for most of my life. My insurance wasn't connected to my job so when I put in my two weeks, it wouldn't affect the appointments. So that was another bullet dodged. Now for the things I was dreading the most, calling my boss to get my two weeks.
I liked my boss, it felt like he was the only friend I had. We had become friends through our mutual interest with Stephen King. I had been reading a re-printed version of Pet Sematary when he commented on it. We had spent the utmost of an hour talking about Stephen King. He had mentioned his wife, and the rest was a blank of gossip and shit talk. We had mentioned so much, we had learned so much, and he was someone that I could consider a friend.
I stared at the phone, it was the only time of called him professionally. I got his phone number the same day, we called, texted, and Facetime. A few weeks after that I was invited to his house with his wife and children. His children were so young that the third time I came over they started calling me "auntie". My god, I loved those kids. They seemed to light up my life, along with the rest of his family. His wife was the sweetest thing ever. Running her own candle business and still having time to make food for her husband and children.
When I was over at their house, I had seen a healthy relationship. She would cook and he would clean, while she put the kids to bed. He would come up after they brushed their teeth and read a story together and kissed them goodnight. I was in awe of their family dynamic and how they loved each other and their kids.
I knew that I would be able to leave this world and earth knowing that at least 5 people would love me. (or at the very least missing me).

Dialing the number I start pacing around my apartment in stress. Walking back and forth in the walkway I am weighing the pros and cons of hanging up and going higher. By the time I decide to do it, the receptionist Barbra is on the line. Me and Barbra hadn't known each other, but we coexisted. She was nice and motherly. Reminding me to drink and eat.

"This is Barbra, how can I help"

After hearing this voice for six years, telling me to eat and drink, it almost felt that I was telling her that I was ending it all.

I froze, for at least a good 2 minutes

"Hello, hon? Are you there?"

"Yeah, hi Barbra"

"Oh, Hi hon, what can I do for you"

"Can you connect me to Don, please"

"Of course, but I thought you had his number already"

"This is more professional, than personal"

"Alright just give me a minute, there we go! Have a good day, dear!"

'Yeah...You to Barbra"

As the distorted elevator music plays in my right ear all I can think about is Barbra. How sweet she is and how much I am going to miss her. The way she waved me over and made sure I ate.

Don+family

Barbra

Now I have at least 6 people that I hope will miss me.

As the phone finally connects I hear Don say "Ahoy, hoy!" A joke that me and him had made.

It was last year around August, I came over for beers. It was around 7:00 pm when the Simpson came on and we heard that. Being so drunk is the funniest thing ever. Don decided that's how he would answer any type of phone call.

"Hey, Don..."

"Hey! How are you? Why are you calling from here?"

"I am doing...alright, but I needed to talk to you professionally"

"Ohhh, you need me to play Mr. Big and mean boss, okay!"

"Yeah, I was wondering about...about putting in my two weeks."

"Wait, what!"

"Yeah, I know..."

"Why? I thought you liked it here"

"I do! I love it here, but I got moved to a new district in New York"

"Fuck...really?"

"Yeah, I tried talking to them, but the pay was higher and they would help with a unit until I could pay by myself"

"No, I get it...Inflation is a bitch, well I'll send you the paperwork then."

"Hey, look I could come over for dinner at one point before I move...would that be okay"

"Yeah, that would be great! Text me later and we can work it out later!"

"Alright, bye Don"

I didn't wait for him to say bye back. I had to hang up. I felt the frozen waffles that I had eaten coming up.

Running to the bathroom I nearly tripped over my cat. I finally made it to the bathroom and nearly opened the toilet seat and lid, but I made it.

Goddamn it…
I felt so bad about lying to my friend, or who I considered a friend.
Finally coughing up the rest of my food, I flush the toilet. Watching the water circle around, I wish I could follow it down. I wish I could be like water, just flowing around a molecule in the middle of millions of the same molecules. How nice that would be following the rest of the water, lost in the world until it ends. Without realizing it I started to feel tears roll down my cheeks. I had no clue why I was crying, there was no reason to.
Standing up, my knees felt weak. I stumbled back and bumped into the towel rack. Regaining my equilibrium I take a single step to the sink. Leaning over the sink I was my face and grabbed my toothbrush. I started to scrub my teeth with such aggression that I started to bleed. When I spit the toothpaste fuzz out it was a creamy pink color. Gulping water, I spit out the water to the same pinkish color as well as a fuzz. I washed my mouth 3 more times to get the residue of blood out. Each time I rinsed out the water burned and fizzed my raw gums. Squatting down, my elbows and forearms on the counter. I started to sob, I could then feel the softness of my cats rubbing against my legs. They were trying to comfort me by using their soft fur and the purring that I love on me. It did work.
I felt myself lose the small balance that I had fallen backward on the floor. My gray cat jumps out from behind me as I land on my ass. Crying into my hands with my knees to my chest. My cats are still surrounding me. 30 minutes after crying, I fell asleep on the ground.

Chapter 5

May 20th

It had been around two days since science decided to kill me. I woke up in my bed, with my three cats surrounding me. Laying my head back down on my pillow I look lovingly at them. How cute they were and how loveable their faces were. I knew that I would leave them in with Don and his family. I had left town awhile before my decision, and while there Don offered to take in my cats. I was a spectacle at first, their family had 3 dogs, and all different breeds. Nonetheless, Don assured me that he would take care of my cats and keep them safe. When I returned to pick up my cats I had seen them sleeping with the dogs and Don's kids on their couch. My cats woke up to the sounds of my adoration towards them.

Looking back on the memory of that scene the cats, dogs, and kids were all snuggling. Looking at my cats I knew they would fit in just right.

I got up around 30 minutes later, I had put on my best genes and a Nirvana shirt. I was meeting with my attorney to decide where everything was gonna go. This wouldn't be long as I didn't have a lot. Waiting in the office of my estate planning attorney I look around at the amount of people in that office. Most were old people with liver spots and old bones. Walkers, canes, and IV drips all around me. There, a woman and man closest to the desk. Watching as she had IV drips and a head cover. I could make out that she had cancer, watching all these people slowly dying from sickness. I had the sickness inside, and I wanted to be gone.

Hearing my name being called, I got thrown back into waiting for my therapist. I shivered when I went back with the secretary. I sit on a chair that has cushions that aren't very soft.

"Hello, Ms.Kyrin"

"Hi. um, I am here to talk about my will"

"Oh! Really? I would have never guessed, but what do you need?"

I see the curiosity on his face about why the hell I am here, but he never asks. I was super glad about that. I had told them about sending the rest of my savings and life insurance to be sent to certain charities. As well as having my cats sent to Don's house. My more valuables like my jewelry would be gifted to Don's wife. My art supply would be sent to his son. As well as my book collection being sent to his daughter. Finally, all my camera equipment was sent to Don. For my sister, it would be my fine china collection that's from our grandmother. After all that, I was able to leave.

Sitting down on the bench right outside the building I can look around at the scenery. Hearing the birds in the trees and seeing the mundane people walk their dogs. Smelling the flowers around me, yellow, pink, and purple. I felt content at this moment closing my eyes and hearing and smelling everything. Finally opening my eyes I see the sun glare, flinching back and raising my hand above my eyes for shade.

Standing up I walk back to my car. Sitting inside waiting for it to cool down a little. I decided to just get some Chinese food. I knew Once I got home I wasn't getting up for a while.

When going to the same place over and over they finally knew what I was going to get. I got chicken fried rice and sweet and sour chicken. When getting my order I never listened to the price. I know exactly what it is, 15.78 dollars. I just pull out my card and pay, not even getting my receipt anymore.

Again autopilot

Sitting on the counter I pet my cats that are crossing in front of me. I eat with a spoon, I can't work chopsticks that well. I have the chicken on the side of me, with Chick-fil-A sauce. I don't know why I like doing this, just for some reason. I am using all paper plates at this point. A while ago I gave away my cutlery so I didn't have to deal with it.

Watching my cats slowly and deliberately move around the island. I loved watching them do these mundane things around the house. It brings me such joy to watch them do such mundane things. They bring such joy to me that I know Don's family will feel as well.

Chapter 6

May 23rd

Waking up around 7:30 in the morning was the best. It was one of the nicer things that came with paid leave. Sitting up I see my cats in the won cuddle pile. I look around my bedroom, realizing the poor state it's in. I should probably clean it, but at the same time, I don't want to spend my last minutes cleaning up. Finally deciding to get up and be productive, I throw my legs over the edge of my bed and slip into my slippers. I am always surprised with how soft these ten-dollar slippers are.

Lifting my body weight I walk over to the coffee machine that I have had for nearly 5 years. I always joked that I would be buried with that coffee machine. How weird to look at death as a joke when you plan to end it all.

While the coffee was brewing I fed my cats. While the days have been getting closer and closer, I have become more lenient with my cats. Letting them do some more things and getting away with it. It was a lot nicer to not worry that much. Grabbing my done coffee I walk back to the room. I lean on the door frame and sigh. If there was ever a room that I wanted to end it all it would be this one. And I should not allow my death room to be this dirty.

I take a big swig of coffee and set it up on the dresser. I first deal with the clothes that are on the floor. Dirty and clean, whatever, just wash them all. I had to go on three trips for all the clothes. I decided to start dusting around the apartment.

Most of the reasons that the apartment looked too grimy was because it was old, and the uncleanliness. There were, no janitors, but they would do routine cleanings for the lobby and just drop off packages for the residence.

Finally finishing up I get my clothes out and fold (or hang) all of them. Finally being opened to the bed I move and rip off all the sheets.

Back to the washing machine

Again…

Something I never understood with my OCD was how I loved order but refused to order my movement. My movement wasn't ever that important to me, and what I did. While thinking of it now, the fact that I don't like repeating movements verbatim might be a part of My OCD.

Looking back around at the room it looked so different. Still musty and old, but of a coziness to it than before. It had a sense of soul now. It was probably the open curtains and mess cleaned up, but I started to look at the apartment with a new feeling.

Moving around the room I feel a sense of comfort, but that suddenly disappeared when I saw a specific photo. It was me and my *best friend*. When that picture was taken was the year we graduated from Iowa State College. We had dark blue graduation gowns on, our hats nowhere to be seen. (I had lost my mind, turns out that my friend held on to it for all these years). We only made funny faces when taking pictures together. It was a solemn feeling. As my depression got worse, we disconnected.

Thinking about it, it would be nice to call or see her. I still have her number saved as a favorite on my phone. I had been too much of a pussy to call her, I always backed out last minute.

We had a falling out when I found out I had infertility, I didn't tell her. She was so excited for me to have kids with my boyfriends. Nonetheless, I didn't tell her, I was afraid of how she would react. Regardless, my sister kept being more and more annoyed with not telling her how the process was going. Even though I was at fault I did hold a grudge for her to keep pestering me, and not having any time. She's my sister, she should know when to talk to me about someone.

Finally gaining some courage how to contact my sister. I grabbed my phone, it had been so long that her number was plenty at the bottom of my 'recent contacts'. After what felt like ages upon ages of scrolling, I finally came across her contact.

"Clone Wars"

My father loved certain sci-fi movies and one series was Star Wars. After watching these movies for years and years we had come up with a multitude of inside jokes; one being calling each other clones.

I fondly remember this as I click the call button. Now I stand in the idle of my apartment with my cats rubbing on my ankles, wallowing in anxiety.
`Bringg`
`Bringg`
`Bringg`
'I feel like I am gonna have a heart attack' I think to myself. My heart is beating so fast, it's not natural. I am surely gonna die to the speed of my heart.
`Bringg`
`Bringg`
`Brin-`
"Hello?"
The feeling of my blood freezing overwhelms me. I haven't heard this voice in nearly 4 years.
She sounded so lively, so pure. The same way I remembered my sister.
"Hello?"
"..."
"Look, if you not gonna say anything then I am hanging up"
"No…wait please"
"Who is this?..."
"It's me…"
"Who exactly is me?"
"I swear to god if this is a prank-"
"Clone Wars!...it's me Clone Wars…"
"Penelope?"
"Yeah…Hi"
"Wh-why are you calling"
"I was wondering…if you…"
"Yes….?
"I was wondering if you wanted to meet up…"
"Oh, you want to see... me?"
"Yeah I do…do you want to"
"Do I Want To? Yes! I want to see you dumbass!"
Before the call was layered with tension coming from both parties, but after that smiling finite little joke, we both seemed more happy. That's what I loved about my sister. She was always able to light up someone in a stupid or meaningful way. That's why she was made out to be a good mother. My sister, Lily, always took care of me. And the few times I met her kids I could tell that she was using experiences from me to help them. This is why it surprised me even more when she wanted me to have kids.
"Look I have to go, Sarah just threw her cup of milk on her brother. I'll text you when I can, okay?"
Lily was rushing to get that sentence out, I could her feet shuffling against the hardwood floor, urging the rest of her body to move. Also, I could hear the sound of her children in the background, and her husband trying to de-escalate the situation, this made me smile.
"Yeah, that would be okay, say 'hi to the family for me okay? Love you…Bye"
"Love you, bai!"

Hanging up the phone I let out a sigh of relief. That had gone better than expected with calling her. I fell back onto the couch, which awoke something inside of me. I started to giggle and feel all giddy inside.
God, how I am gonna miss my sister…

Chapter 7

May 30th

The time spent between now and the call with my sister was long. In this time gap, I had been spending more time outside. I picked up reading art history books, again. I have always read them when I was a kid. They were my favorite. My father used to say, "One day you're gonna' turn into a painting' '. I would always giggle at that. Dinner with my sister and her family was scheduled for tomorrow, I am nervous but excited. I can't wait to see my nephews, after the phone call with my sister I rejected not sending anything to her family. Then I remembered something that happened a while ago. When we first led our father into the nursing home where he currently resides, we talked about his will. I said that I would take his fine china and his old 50s artwork that he held dear. When asking my sister about what she wanted I remembered her solemn face. It was pale and sunken as if she had not slept for the past week. Lily was so bright before when we had gotten breakfast together, now she was completely different.
Lily talked about how she could never have something from anyone's will. That having reminders of them would break her more than death. She started to sob quietly, then loudly. It broke my heart, I walked over and hugged her, it was the first time I ever hugged her. I had my eyes, trying not to ruin the moment even more with the discomfort present in my face. The only reason I realized that she started to cry into my chest was when I felt a wet, cold patch on my lower chest. I knew I was supposed to comfort her, but I couldn't. I froze. Lily didn't notice that, she was too deep in her feelings. Taking deep breaths I try to relax but whenever Lily's ragged breaths reach my ears I lose my balance. We left there in tears and discomfort, not what we had planned for.
Knowing this information, a letter would suffice for her. As I sit against an old oak tree, I think of what to say in the letter. Maybe something along the lines of how it wasn't her fault. How do I know this is best for me, I know that this was selfish and I am sorry.
It should be something like that, that would be good.
Now I can only think about this scene of my sister on her knees with her hand over her mouth. Hot tears ran down her face, her face red hot from the lack of oxygen. Her husband tries to comfort her by hugging her, but it doesn't work, she is too distraught. Her two sons are in the back, unable to understand why

their mom is crying this hard. I can imagine the letter on the floor in front of my sister, teardrops running over the ink.
I know that this might be a bad idea, but I don't want my sister to blame herself. It was never truly her fault. Standing up I light a cigarette, I had given up smoking when I met my boyfriend and I didn't get back into it until I was sure about committing suicide. I figured I was going to die in two weeks, so why not? I head back to my apartment, the world seems so bright outside. Colorful and full of happiness, but then I walk into my apartment building. The world is now damp and sad.
Finally getting into my apartment from the depressing world that is the hallway. I sat down at my desk, my body had become more used to this seat now more than ever. I had been starting to sleep at my desk recently (and coach), and I wanted my room to be perfectly pristine for when the time came.
Getting out paper and a pen, I harness my best handwriting.

Dear Lily,

When you get this you will already know the news. It's not your fault. This was a very hard decision, but it's what I need. I can't bear to live in this world anymore, there's too much pain. I love you so much, I am sorry that you will have to bear the burden of my death. The one thing I will ask of you is to take care of Dad, and see him more regularly please, he talks so fondly of you.

Love, Your clone

One thing I didn't expect is how easily the words fell onto the page. It was almost as if the words wrote themselves, they were almost to go to be from my mind, but it was perfect. I read over the letter a multitude of times, unbeknownst to me I started to cry, hard. I could feel myself shaking, and the ability to breathe slowly slipping away from me. Falling over on the desk I started loudly sob, like a goddamn baby. What was interesting was that I was crying so hard that I fell asleep.
After waking up it was around 5 at night. Only slept for about an hour, not too bad. Getting up I walked over to the fridge, as well as getting outside more, I started to cook more. It was nice to be in the kitchen with my playlist on, dancing to my heart's content. I cooked some salmon and broccoli. The kitchen smells delicious, and I also cook a pecan pie, the last time I visited the kids, they loved this. They said mine was the best with a little lisp on their pronunciation of "th", so cute. I am so excited for tomorrow.

Chapter 8

May 31st

I woke up nice and early to get ready (off the couch). Deciding that this is important, I put a lot more work into myself than I normally would when getting ready. I used my best shampoo and shaved my legs. Blew dried my hair and used makeup, it was good 5 years early when I bought this.

We had decided that I would show up at noon and we would decide when to leave. Shaking, I was so excited! My sister was making our favorite childhood meal, five-cheese pasta. It was simple, meaning it was one of the only things our dad could make without burning the house down. Nonetheless, it had grown on us even into adulthood. I could already imagine the smell and taste. Lily's version of the pasta was always better than my dad's. This was a secret we promised to keep because it would break my dad's heart, until a fight. Me, Lily, and Dad were all in a fight and I screamed about how I preferred Lily's pasta to his. It shut us all up quickly. I was so overstimulated by the fighting that once those words left my lips, I started to cry. And I mean CRY! It sucked in the moment, but it was something that I could look back on with a laugh. Because that was the worst thing I could physically say to my dad.

I got into the car, this is when my anxiety hit me. Finally, I realized how personal I and my sister were going to get, and what I was going to have to explain to her. Deciding that I would cross the bridge when I came to it, I started to car. It was around 11:20 a.m I've always been one to be earlier than prepared. I hope my sister remembers this and tries to accommodate it.

I pull up in front of her house. It's 11:50 p.m. close to noon. Looking around the house it was different from the last time I visited. Last time it was a 50's pinkish color, not it changed to a robin's egg blue. This was the boy's favorite color combined, light blue and turquoise. The garden changed a little as well, there were a lot more yellow flowers than last time, and most of them were tulips. Lily's favorite flower are tulips and her favorite color is yellow.

Cute!

Getting out of the car, it was 11:56 a.m. I walk over to the door, it's a double door with, a white door frame and white door, and it fits nicely. Knocking on the door, it's the "two-bit' knock. A little plain but fun to do for us. Waiting around I hear fast, little steps running around the house, screaming "Auntie! Auntie!" I have to giggle at that. I hear footsteps stop at the door but then continue with a jumping noise. That's when I hear the unmistakable sounds of heels clicking on the hardwood floors.

As the doorknob turns, the world slows down. My heart is beating in my ears, I can feel my blood flowing in my body as I watch the crack in the door grow more and more. That's when I finally saw her, my sister. She looks just how I remembered, but somehow even more beautiful.

Lily had little auburn hair that seemed to glow in the day. With lovely hazel eyes, but they seemed gray in the winter.

"CLONE!"

"Hi, Lily…"

I am pretty awkward as she hugs me, but soon I revel in the hug. Wrapping my arms around her I feel this warm feeling in my chest that I haven't felt in any way. I wrap my arms around her tighter and tighter, I fear that if I don't hug her tight enough then she'll leave.

"Woah, tiger, I am gonna stop breathing if you keep squeezing me like that!"

"Sorry…I am just evicted to see you."

"Ditto, but anyway I am sure the kids are happy too! Ain't that right?!"

"YEAH!"

Just then I get two six-year-olds hugging onto my calves. Kneeling I take them both in my arms and squeeze as tight as I physically can.

"Auntie! We have grown so much, see!"

They pull me to the doorway where I can see the markings in pencil. 4'5, 4'11, 5'0, and 5'2.

"I know I almost didn't recognize you!"

"Liar! Yes, you did!"

Their faces are scrunched up in laughter. They run back to the kitchen to talk to their dad.

"Well are you ready"

"Yeah…I guess"

Stepping into the house I am immediately met with familiar warmth. Her home always had a very warm palette, a beachy home. We walk over to the dining table, a nice mahogany color with benches except on the end with two chairs. Lily's husband sits at the end, the boys sit on his left side, and me and my sister sit on his right side.

The table is filled with chicken, mac & cheese, broccoli, and mashed potatoes. It smelled delicious, I wished that I would cook like this more. I brought out my pecan pie early and it was sitting in the warming oven.

After a few words of appreciation, we all dug in. With the warmth in my heart and my stomach being filled with delicious food, I felt as if I could die right here and be completely content with my life.

After dinner, we washed up, and I was told to sit my ass down after wanting to help with the plates.

Me and Lily's husband, Jason, were talking about the world of creativity. Jason was a muralist who worked under his management. It was interesting always talking to him, he held this level of authority that seemed to just vanish when you got him comfortable. We kept talking through eating my pie, which everyone complimented.

After some more talking and playing, my sister took me outside to talk.

Chapter 9

May 31st

I am sitting outside with my sister on her second porch. Rich Fucks.
Lily made me black tea. I like black tea but not excessively. Like I can drink a few sips of it, but I can't drink a whole cup of it. Most of the time I'll just hold it and wait until they leave so I can pour it out.
Where their house is they have a field behind the house. There are lots of flowers and wild animals. The animals are always domestic, like bunnies, deer, sheep goats, and chickens because of the farm next to the house. I feel the breeze on my face and hair. I can feel my baby hairs flowing in the wind.
"So…what did you want to say"
I can feel the awkwardness in the air, you could cut the tension with the knife. I have to stay confident, this is the last time that I talk to her.
Taking in a deep breath, I start:
"I wanted to talk about what happened"
"Alright, I'll let you speak…"
"Alright, so me and Jackson broke up, we broke up after I found out I was infertile. The reason I didn't tell you about it was that I was embarrassed, I gave so much hope that me and him were gonna work and have a kid, but…I felt so sad about what I failed to do that I ended up distancing myself, and I am sorry"
Stopping, I take a shaking breath in. I didn't even realize that I was on the verge of crying until I stopped. The breeze is blowing, drying out my eyes, I wait for her to leave. Or at the very least just say that I was right in not telling her.
Looking over I am met with empathy, Lily has her hand over her heart, her shoulders sunken.
"Oh, Penelope"
Lily reaches over and hugs me, I am still holding the cup of black tea in my hand. This urge to hug her back rose in my chest. I set the cup on the table and immediately reached over to hug her back. I start crying, purply sobbing into my sister's shoulder.
"Shhh, it's okay…thank you for telling me… I would never think any less of you, especially something you can't control. Thank you for telling me this, it must be hard"
I started to sob more when she said that, finally feeling accepted.
I slowly lean back to gain composure, I take a look back at the cup of black tea, I already drank my fill but the crying made my throat dry. Taking the cup in my

hand, I can see the tear marks in my reflection. Taking a sip I close my eyes and sit to feel the breeze.

"May I ask a few questions, please"

Giving her a nod, she continues,

"Do you still have the house?"

"No, we sold it after about a year"

"Oh, are you still in contact with him?"

"No, after we found out and the year before we sold the house we just drifted apart, and once we made the breakup official, he left with a coworker of his"

"Asshole"

I heard her whisper that under their breath, I didn't say anything about it. Technically it was both our faults. Neither of us reached out to help one another, but Lily didn't need to know that. We would never see him again so what's the point?

"Thanks for not judging me…I was scared as you are a mother yourself"

"No, no, no I could never."

Looking over at her, I smile and lean in to rest my forehead on hers.

"How bout we go inside"

I didn't say anything, but I didn't have to. We had that kind of sister speak. Where we could just tell based on the feeling of what was happening. Lily stands up first, grabbing my hand. She pulls me to stand up with her.

As I stand I feel as if 50 pounds have been lifted off my shoulders. Finally, standing in the presence of my sister I don't feel any awkwardness or stress. All I feel now is happiness.

Chapter 10

June 1st

I have seven days left before my death. And being honest with myself, I have never been happier.

Today I am meeting with my therapist for the last time. I am quite excited, even if most exercises didn't work, my therapist was nice.

Watch as other therapists and psychiatrists come to get their patients. When I would sit here I would always wonder what other people were thinking. Most were on their phone or computers, but there would be that one person who wasn't. I would be curious about what they feel, are they nervous, excited, or neutral?

But now sitting here I am met with a revelation of how I feel.

Clam

That's how I feel, I feel calm with a small dose of anxiety. The room is more sanitary. Looking at the room objectively, the room is similar to a suburban house.

In the distance, I see Ms. Amber. She seems to glow in the midday sun, something I have never seen before. Seeing Ms. Amber face to face in this new light, I only now recognize her beauty. Her dark auburn skin and dark tight curly hair. She looks like a goddess.

"Hello, Ms. Amber"

"Hello, Penelope"

She reaches out her hand, I take it in with gratitude.

"Well let's head to my room and get started, okay?"

Nodding I follow her into her room, I know my way but I find it more respectful to follow her. Finally getting to her office, I look around. Her choices in decor always made quite…shifted. But now, knowing this would be the last time I would see the office, I could finally enjoy it.

"So how have you been, hon?

"Honestly, really good, I've been a lot better!"

"That's..great! What has changed?"

"Well, I haven't had any nightmares, I reconnected with my sister and I started to cook more and more!"

As I talk I reach over and grab a mint off the top of the pile. Even unwrapping the mints I could tell Ms. Amber was writing something down. Taking the mint into my mouth I taste chocolate, I hadn't realized it but my face must have brightened.

"You like?"

"Very much so, what are these?"

"Just some generic type from the store."

"Well, it's nice!"

"Good, anyway have you been taking your medication daily"

I pause, I haven't been taking any medication. It's just sitting on my sink.

"Yeah…"

I am positive she can tell my hesitant answer but I don't care.

"Alright, how are the cats?"

Before I found these mundane questions pretty annoying, but now I am pretty awed that she knows.

"Oh, their good, you know being little shits but so cute while doing it"

"I get that, my little wiener dog is so annoying but he's so cute"

Giggling at that I reach over and grab another mint, there are good

"How's your father?"

"I am not entirely sure, I am visiting him in and few days but I haven't been called or anything"

"Well I guess that's good"

As I look at the clock I realize we have been talking for 20 minutes, nearly done with the sension. Wow, I never realized time went that fast. Ms. Amber noticed that I was in awe of the clock.

"Times flies when you're having fun"

"That's very corny, I hope you know that"

It's a minute of silence, I think that I went a little too far. Just safer than I thought I would hear her start to laugh. As she laughed it just hit me that I had never heard her laugh. It's so beautiful.

Finally, the time came to a close after some more talking. Getting up I walk to the door when I hear Ms. Amber's heels behind me. This was the first time she would have ever walked me out. As we walk down the hall, we sit in a comfortable silence. Only the sound of her heels hitting the shiny hardwood floors. I can fear each time as the air grows harder when we cross in front of the AC.

When finally reached the door, we faced each other. Glancing up into her eyes I see some sympathy. 'Does she know?'

Stupid thought but it almost felt like she could tell that this was the last time we would see each other.

"I'll see you later"

"Bye, Ms. Amber"

Walking over to the elevator I can feel my steps quicken in pace. Getting into the elevator I start pressing the button quickly. I don't know why but I feel like I am worried for no reason.

Getting into the elevator I let out a sigh of relief. Jumping I feel my phone vibrate in my pocket. Getting my phone out I see it Don, I realize that we haven't talked about dinner yet.

"Heyo!"

Even hearing myself I am surprised with how happy I seem.

"Ahoy-hoy, you sound happy!"

"I got out of a really good therapy session with a therapist, it was nice"

"That's fantastic, anyway me, Jen, and the kids are free tomorrow if you wanna come over"

"Yeah that sounds great, send me the time!"

"Perfect!-Hey! Stop that!"

I can hear their kids screaming in the background, I assume they're playing with the dogs. And if I was right on cue I could hear the dogs barking.

"I'll catch you on the flip side, bye"

"Bye-"

The call ends abruptly causing me to laugh a little. I walk home with a little pep in my step going home. I am so excited to see Don. Walking I stop mid-track to realize that I should cook something for them. Maybe a carrot cake, his wife loves my carrot cake, but the kids don't. Maybe a carrot cake and some chocolate chip cookies for the kids!

Oh, that sounds so good! Alright, I made up my mind! Now onto the store for the ingredients.

Chapter 11

June 4th

Waking up makes me happy. I remembered that I was gonna go to Don's. Walking out I realize that I am gonna have to make a cake and cookies. I feel this weight in my chest about doing this. I am regretting my choice of deciding this. While I didn't even tell them I still felt an obligation to do it. Maybe it's because of my father, my dad always talked about being true to your word. He rammed that into my brain at a very young age. That's one of my core memories. My dad and I are sitting in the living room as he talks about his war stories. Him talking about the loyalty of promises in the war.
Those memories with my father were always a little weird. His stories hold memories of violence but it was such a sweet moment together.
Deciding that I would make it nonetheless, I pull out my phone while sighing. When ordering the food I felt the hit of reality. Just now it hit me that this was the last time I was going to face Don. Same with my sister and my father, I am never going to see them again. Well, last impressions are just as important as first impressions.
Waiting on the groceries I turn on the TV, turning on 'Independence Day'. This movie is old, but it's good. It's nosologic, most of my favorite actors are in this. Will Smith and Jeff Goldblum, for the same reason I like 'Aliens', for Sigourney Weaver. It's about the 20-minute mark in the movie when the food arrives. Everything has almost the same ingredients, besides the obvious. Grabbing the ingredients I decided to make the cake first. The cake will take an hour while the cookies will take around 30 minutes. So, I'll be able to get cookies in around the half mark of the cake. Works out well for my time management and getting there with hot gifts. Once mixed with all the ingredients for the carrot cake I spray the pan and pour the mix in. When pouring in the mix I realize that I have to make the icing. Deciding that I will make it later, I start with the cookies. There's

something about baking that always clams me. I think it's how my brain just focuses on one thing. There is so much that goes into baking that you forget everything. Your brain is so focused on the measurements and mixing that you block everything else out. It's like your brain is running a marathon and winning is getting the thing in the oven.

After the cookies are in the oven I take a moment to breathe. Looking at the sink, it is covered in dishes and I decide to leave it for later. Grabbing the sugar and the butter I start to make the icing for the cake. Once finished, I start my least favorite part of baking; the icing. I find this to be messy and hard. The icing can fall off, and the heat of the cake can ruin it. It takes me about 15 minutes before I finally say 'fuck it' and go for the rustic type of icing job. I barely put any icing on it and called it done. I grab a container and put the cake in as well as the cookies. Finally, I finished and it was just the perfect time to go over.

I finish the drive to Don's place. I stay in the car for a few minutes, I keep taking looks out of the window. This place holds so many memories and I have felt so much love here that I am conflicted about my feelings. I look around at the yard, full of toys and dog toys. Almost like a hallucination, I can see the kids playing with the dogs and Don watching them from the porch. Leaning my head back on the seat, I let out a breath that I didn't know I was holding. Finally, I get out of the car and grab the treats. It feels like slow motion as I make my way up to the porch and ring the doorbell. As slow as it was to walk up to the door, it was so fast how Don's wife opened the door.

"Oh, Penelope! How lovely to see you!"

I nod and reciprocate the same affection to her in a similar tone.

"Kids! Don! Look who's here. Can I help with the stuff?"

Before even responding Don's wife already had the cake in hand and walked to the kitchen. I hear the sounds of the two kids running in from the backyard. I see Don's daughter who has on a blue dress and hair in ponytails. His son runs in with jeans shorts and a dinosaur tee shirt. His daughter was 7 and his son was 4. Getting on one of my knees I embrace them. Scence they were a little small. I was still able to pick them up like I normally would. I swung them around as I heard them laugh and giggle, playfully calling out my name. Finally putting them down I can hear their dad walk in and tell them to help their mother. Finally getting to see Don after this time, it felt like years. I embraced him, for probably the last time.

"It's so nice of you to do this, you didn't need to bring anything"

"You say that now, but once you get your hands on my carrot cake you gonna thank me"

"Yeah you're right..come in"

Getting in I sit down at the table watching as Don's wife puts the final plate of food on the table. I should have paid more attention to what they were putting on the table, or even what I was putting on my plate. I just wanted to enjoy the last time I saw them. The kids sit across from me and their mother, while Don sits at the head of the table. We all have a hearty meal filled with life and laughter. Once done we all help clear the table (even though I was told I didn't need to). Finally, me and Don sit out on the porch watching the kids and the dogs while his wife finishes up.

"So, what do you think about moving to New York?"

"Huh?- Oh! Oh yeah, I think it's cool"

I forgot that I told Don that specific lie, about why I was putting my two weeks in.
"You sounded confused when I asked."
"Oh yeah, it feels so surreal that I am moving there that it almost feels unreal."
Don hummed in agreement but I don't think he believed me in the long run. We
kept talking for hours until it was dark out. It didn't feel that long but whatever.
Once we were at the door so I could go home I felt all of my emotions hit me all
at once. I leaned down to hug the kids and started to cry, and it was hard. I
heard this daughter turn her head and ask why I was crying. They were
devastated when they found out that I was supposed to move away, and they
started to cry all the same. Finally standing up I collect myself and Hug his wife
and Finally Don. We only exchanged a few 'goodbyes' as I walked to my car.
Finally, I decide to write Don a letter as well, again I find myself sitting at my
desk with a pen and paper.

Dear Don,

*This was a personal decision that held a lot of thought. Nonetheless, I want
to thank you for being my friend. I would be in a much darker place if I
didn't have you and your family by my side. I am sorry that I am leaving
you, but I hope you hold me dear along with the memories that you have
with me.*

Love, Penelope

*(P.s. I swear if something happens to my cats I will come back and haunt
you)*

Getting done with the letter I put it in an envelope and put it on my bed next to
Lily's letter.

Chapter 12

June 6th

Today I am seeing my dad. My father is 79 years old and is in assisted living.
About 5 years ago he was diagnosed with lung cancer (all those damn smokes)
He was very into the idea of assisted living and I don't blame him at all. I mean
my father lived by himself and two kids for most of his life.
My mother, who I didn't know, left when I was 2. My father didn't know what to
do with what he was handed. He worked on construction sites, and he often
worked very late. I can remember my father rushing for the first couple of years
of my life. Being busy with his job and kids there was barely any downtime.
Once me and my sister hit 12 and were able to walk to and from school he
relaxed. You could see the relief he had when we both graduated from 8th
grade and went to high school.
When driving home I always get a nervous feeling in my stomach. It is almost
painful when going to the home. There is almost a painful air surrounding the
home. It makes me queasy going there sometimes, completely sick to my
stomach. Most of the time, when I went home after visiting him I would throw up.
Driving home, I get a sudden memory of when I told my dad about my infertility
and my breakup.
I was sitting facing the window that opened up to a field in the back. My dad and
I just watched the wind blow the trees and watched the shadows. I looked at his
face through the reflection of the glass. My chest was heavy with dread. I kept
facing the window, carefully planning out how to go about what I was saying.
"Dad?"
"Hm?..."
My father was never one for words, more comfortable with silence.
"I have something….I have something to tell you."
I noticed his eyes glance at me through the window.
"Me and my boyfriend broke up…and"
I felt my breath hitch up as I thought about it. My father liked my boyfriend, they
liked the same things. My father also liked the thought of us having kids.
"And I found out that…that I am..infertile"
I tried to be strong and keep my head high but in the end, I couldn't. My head
dropped down and to the left out of shame. I was staring at the cold, white, and
sanitized floor.
"Hm…."
Once I hear my dad hum in thought I quickly glance back at him. I expected to
see some sort of anger or disappointment, but what I was met with was just a
blank stare.
"I don't think any less of you, muffin"
I can feel his hand reach mine. My dad's hands were always cold, but now they
had warmth. We didn't say anything else at the moment. I didn't say anything
either, the moment didn't need any speaking. After a minute of gathering my
feelings, I scooted next to him and rested my head on him.

As I sit outside of the home I start to think of what's gonna happen when I get inside. What should I say to him? Should I even talk, or should I be just one of those quiet moments that people have?

Saying 'fuck it' I walk to the home and ring the front desk. In the home, they still have some old TVs, some from the 70s I believe. Ms. Carol- a nurse- told me that some of the people who have Alzheimer's like to be familiar with a few things, like the TV model. When I told Dad this he said that it was stupid, it didn't matter what TV it was as long as he watched his shows. After a month there I checked on him and he gave me 5 dollars for being right about the tvs.

Walking over to the table he is in the same spot as we always are. Sitting in a wheelchair with the logo of the home on the back, his head is tilted slightly left. He sits with a cardigan that he got as a welcome home gift after being in the Air Force. He always keeps a chair next to him in case I make a surprise visit and do not tell him.

He's always been a very prepared guy.

Without saying anything I sit by him and stare out the window. It looks the same as last time, it's almost creepy how similar it was. I could feel my dad look at me when I sat down, again after I didn't say anything. As annoyed as he may have seen when you would babble about something, he always did enjoy the noise. After counting to not say anything I hear him clear his throat.

My throat is dry

I can't get anything out.

Reaching over I can feel his shaky, and bony hand on my leg. It's comforting in its way, like when he would give a handshake or a pat on the back instead of a hug or kiss. Almost as if I am transported back, I can smell the roast beef, potatoes, and green beans. It was July of the 80-something. I had made it into the state champion for my writing essay. I was so proud that my eyes were closed from how big my smile was. Once I opened my eyes I saw my father. A big burly man of 6'3 with a wife beater and a pair of jeans on. The light reflects on his back, an ashtray full of cigars and beer. His face is uninterested, bored even. I can feel my smile lower and lower until there is no emotion on my face. I clear my throat, reiterating what I had said before but in a neutral tone. He hummed and got up leaving the room just in time for my arms to fall to my side. My shoulders drop with them and I start to take shallow and quick breaths, trying to not cry. I can feel my stomach cramp into itself and I lean on the table for support. Opening my eyes I stare down at the blue Macleod tartan pattern that is rested upon the table and see water droplets on it. Getting up I wipe my face off in the sink and go up to the bedroom.

When I lay awake at night I remember this.

Now sitting with my father as I plan to kill myself in 2 days, I can't feel the same resentment as I did before. Now, he was just a man, who was my father. An old one who didn't get enough love or recognition from his father and passed it along.

"I would've brought you some banana bread, but the nurses say you can't have more salt"

I don't know why I said it, but it just happened. The most regular conversation that we can have and yet there is still something wrong.

Glancing over at my dad in the window and I see his eyes. Behind the dead stare to the grass, there is something there. Something that I can make out as sorrow. Looking into his eyes and seeing that I feel like he knows.
'He knows what I am gonna do' I think, but then I remember that I am crazy to think that. 'He can't read my thoughts, he has no clue'. I try to calm down but I still can't calm that feeling. It's so weird.
After what feels like an eternity I look back to the grass. It's still the same. All the same, it's gonna be the same when my dad finds out, along with Don and my sister. All the goddamn same.
I don't know how long I was sitting there with my father lost in thoughts, gazing at the ground. Finally snapping out of it I see the major change in the shadows. Checking the time I realize that it's half past 5.
"I should be getting home."
I say that after every visit when I have to or want to leave. Standing up I hear the wood creak. It wasn't that loud but there were ears with a mega blast of sound in my ears. Wincing, I bend down and kiss my father's forehead. He doesn't do anything, for a minute I think he's dead until I see his left hand move. It moved upwards and towards his right shoulder and grabbed at my hand that was resting there. It's a small squeeze but it's noticeable. I walk away making a second stop to the desk.
"Yes?"
The lady at the desk has a high-pitched voice and bubbly tone.
"I need you to hold on to this for my dad"
I was already checked in so they didn't need my name or who I was seeing. Reaching into my pocket I grab the envelope that's in there and hand it to her. I wrote one for my father after I wrote Lily's, it doesn't say much but it does say this:

Dear dad,

My life is complete and I love you, take care

-Penelope

Like I said not much, but it's enough for my dad. Handing the envelope to the lady, she gives me a confused look.
"When should I give him this?"
"After his other daughter, Lily, calls him."
I know immediately she will call him after she calms down and collects her thoughts. Walking out I sit in the car and lean back, sighing I start the car and leave the parking lot on the way to my apartment.
Getting home I flop on the couch and sleep without taking my shoes off.

Chapter 13

June 7th

One day.
That's what is left it is one day.
24 hours of life are left.
Frozen, staring at where the end of my life would occur.
I felt myself leave my body. As an onlooker of a movie screaming at the main character not to do it. But it's not true, it's only me and my thoughts, no one's gonna stop me. Only when I feel my cat's soft fur rub against my leg do I snap out of it. My chest is released from its constraints and I can breathe again. I quickly dart out of the room and close the door, my cat rushing beside me and staring like it could sense something. I walk back to the couch and sit, taking a minute to contemplate what just fucking happened. Reaching out for the remote I grab onto it and put in a movie. I need to be away from these thoughts, the movie that's on is Hobbs& Shaw, a movie about fast and furious characters. I don't care about the franchise but I do like the actors so I decided to put that on one last time.

Chapter 14

June 8th

Today is the day, the day that I die.

Chapter 15

June 8th

I watch the emoji I just sent my sister. A smiley face, with the eyes closed and blushing. And opposite of what I feel. I look at the time
11:23 a.m
June 8th
It's today that I die

Looking over at my apartment I start to think about what's gonna happen to it. My landlord was pretty lenient with decoration, painting walls, or peeling and sticking wallpaper. The leniency of the decoration policy would cause someone to go all out. I like the idea of a woman, and a dog moving in. She's a maximalist and would have those maximalist tiger wallpaper. With some butterfly wallpapers in her room to differentiate. The kitchen would be remolded. Yellow cabinets, a nice change from the blue and green bedroom and living room. The closet would be colorful colors, she would have a large amount of jewelry. She might even post it to the media about her day and outfits. Her dog would be a husky, a sassy one. One that yells and howls when it doesn't get what it wants. But she loves the dog to death, she is a pescetarian but she'll feed the dog all the red meat it needs. The woman will have a boyfriend, someone who's dark-skinned. Some fading tattoos, dreadlocks, and a Y2K style. He would have some back problems. Maybe some joining pain, and she would have diabetes. They would be a match in heaven. Not married, they don't see the reason. The marriage doesn't make the love they have anymore finalized. They have each other and that's all they need.

Or will it be a mother and a child? The mom redoes the office or extra room into the kid's room. She'll take my room. She'll redo the cracking wall paint in my room. Shell does a cream color, and her child a green room. The house will stay neutral with pops of colors from the kid. She'll be a nurse and work late but she'll always keep time for her kids on the days she's not working. They have each other and that's all they need.

Staring at the apartment I think a lot, but I assume that most people won't live here. After finding out a person died here, a lot of people wouldn't buy it. I read the last message from my sister. It's a pink heart with sparkles. I turn my phone off and plug it in. I walk to the kitchen and grab some wet food for the cats. They come running over, I grab their respectful bowl and clank the can on the side. I get so entranced by the sound of the can taping against the bowl that I don't notice that it's already out. Only when I feel my cat rub my ankles do I get out of my head. I do that for the rest of the cats and put the bowls down for them. My tabby jumped down from the counter, and I didn't even notice he was up there. I grab the water fountains for them and turn them on. I walk to the room and close the door. I did this so they wouldn't bother me. I had a stool and noose in there already. Looking around the room I walk over to the bed and flatten it out a little more. I fluff the pillows and slightly move the photographs and the lamp around 20°. I look around one more time and change a few more things. I close the closet doors grab a dust rag and clean the TV. I hold the dust rag in my hand, staring at the grayish dust. I walk out and quickly run to the washing machine. The cats had stopped eating and had left. There is still food there, I know they'll come back. Back in the room, I see all three of my cats. Like they know the reason that I am in there. I stare at them, they're eyes big and round. I watch as they meow and look around the room. I go over and pick them up one by one. Kissing them on the head before dropping them out. I close the door and turn back around. I can hear my cats meowing in desperation. It takes me a minute, I keep turning around to look at the door. I sigh and turn around leaving the room and reaching for the treats. I distract them and run back to the room without them following. I push the door close with my whole body and rest on the door. I lean back up to a standing position. I walk to the stool and noose.

Grabbing the stool I move the stool under the fan. I make sure that I won't bang my head on it. I grab the noose that I already made. I wrap the rope on the metal part of the fan connecting the wooden part to the motor. Getting back down and dropping the noose I realize that if I want this to work I need to find a strong knot to tie. I would use my phone but it's out by the couch and I don't want to deal with the cats again, so I decide on my computer. Searching up my question I understand that the Palomar knot is the best for it. The article does say that it does take a while to master but all I need is to hold my body weight. I grab my laptop and bring it over to the bed and pace gently on the bed. I stand on the stool follow the directions and make sure it's tight. Getting back down I grab my computer turn it off and plug it up. Stand back on the stool and stare at the floor through the noose. I grab around the noose and hold onto it for a good minute. Placing the noose over my neck I sigh and take my last breath. Reach my hand around my neck and tighten the rope around my neck. I kept tightening it so that I could have choked myself while still standing. Taking a breath I already feel the tightness of my throat. Looking down at the floor, I feel like it's over thousands of feet down. Looking up I feel tears in my mind and close them. I push the stool back.

My breath is held on the tip of my tongue but it can't get inside of my lungs. I can feel my eyes burst open and the muscles in my hand tighten. My muscles want to pull on the rope that's around my neck, but I stop them so they're still by my side. I feel drool on my chin and try to swallow, but the rope won't allow it. I start to cough as the spit is pushed back to my lips and onto my chin. Blinking rapidly, my hands go to the rope and hold on to it. I start to feel lightheaded as the blood is being caught by the rope. My legs move rapidly, I can't control them. I realize that I can't control them, my body is in survival mode and won't listen to my brain. It feels like I am throwing up my esophagus. Slowly my muscles lose traction and fall, I close my eyes one last time and everything goes dark.....

My last thought is

"Finally"

-Part 2-

Chapter 16

Lily's POV

June 11th

Everything is quiet as I look around the lawyer's office. I glance at the ground by my left, there's a leather shoe. It's Don's. I only met Dons a little while ago, apparently he's a friend of Penleopes. Based on his looks he seems older than her, by like 3 years. Don is on the tanner side, with freckles and dark hair which is growing gray. I look back at my lap, it is covered in a black dress. The lawyer talks about what Don's family is getting. Her art, camera, cats, books, and jewelry. Finally, the lawyer turns to me as I raise my head. He looks directly into my eyes as he tells me that I left her fine china.

It hurts that she would leave me with so little and Don with so much. But as I think of it, we didn't make it until a week ago. Don was there more and a better emotional outlet for her. Well only so good because she still killed herself. The lawyer keeps a neutral face as he looks at the document again while stating what she would do with her money. I smile at finding out what she decided to do with it. She was always a good person, it showed with the cats that she had. They were runts, all from different litters and unwanted, but my sister and her big heart had her bringing them in. As the lawyer concludes the session he makes a final statement, that we all have letters to read. Walking out I see my husband there with our two boys. I can feel it harder and harder to hold back tears. I turn my head away to not cry from looking at my boys. Don is by his family, he is on one knee. He had each hand on one of his kid's shoulders, I assume he's telling them what they get. I watch the girl start to cry, as the boy's face scrunches up like he's going to. Don's face moves up to look at his wife and she puts her hand over her mouth. He looks back at the kids and hugs them.

I look back over to my boys and walk over. I know they didn't have the best relationship with their aunt as we didn't see her often, but they loved her. I hold their faces in each hand, I lick my lips and sigh.

"Aunt Pee Pee died, and we're gonna have to have a funeral"

"What…?"

We had told the kids that something had happened to Penelope but we didn't say what until now. I can feel my chest shake as my eyes fill with tears.

"Aunt Pee Pee died two days ago and she left us something."

"But…"

I look at my husband as the twins try to make sense. He turns them around and kneels to talk to them. I take a tissue out of my pocket and hold it to my nose as I sniffle. That's when I feel a hand on my shoulder, it's Don's.

Don's POV

After telling the kids what they got from Penelope I turn to look at her sister. She looks like Penelope in a few ways, the same nose and mouth. Turning back around I grab my wife's cheek and kiss her, mumbling that I'll be back. The couple steps that take me to get over to her sister feels like a hike. When reaching her I can hear her sniffle and I contemplate if I even say anything. I tap her on her shoulder, she turns her eyes watery.

"You're Peneleope's sister right?"

Stupid question but she nods nonetheless that I am correct.

"Lily?"

She nods again.

I sigh as I decide on what to say. I and Penelope have had quite a few conversations about family problems. Like me with my father and her with her sister. Finally, I decided on what to say.

"Me and your sister talked a lot about our family problems"

I can see her face scrunch up about what I said. I take another minute before starting again.
"I would talk about my father, and she would talk about you."
Looking into Lily's eyes I could see that she was either going to walk away or cry or slap me. But luckily I finish before any of that happens.
"And the only difference was that she loved you, cared, and appreciated you."
Lily's eyes widen slightly before removing the tissue from her nose and sniffling again. I take this as I sign that she likes what she's hearing.
"If she was ever annoyed at something you did it was always followed by a 'But, she's…' one night-"
I let out a scuff of a laugh before telling her.
"She told me one night that you were her inspiration to get into TV. She told me about how you used to do performances and she was backstage. There was a sparkle in her eyes that I haven't seen anywhere else when talking about you on that stage."
I keep my smile as I watch Lily grow her own. She licks her lips and tells me,
"I was shit in those"
Standing there I tilt my head to catch her eyes that are starting at her right shoe.
"She didn't think so"
Mine and her head raise simultaneously. Finally, I see her actual face. And my gaze lowers to my hand that's in my pocket.
"What should we do about the letters?"
I ask looking back up at her, she seems to realize what I am talking about and pauses. She thinks for a minute before looking back up at me.
"I'm gonna go to my father and tell him the news, but I think it might be better if we read them at our times."
I stare at the linoleum floors. Nodding taking in the information and agrees that it would be easier to read it by ourselves.
"What about the funeral, what are we gonna do for that?" I ask this out of the blue for no reason.
I keep staring at the floor even when I hear Lily's hum as she thinks about what to do. I keep my head down, seeing Lily's hand leave my peripheral.
"Well I would offer to do the funeral arrangements by myself, but I would assume that you would know more about what Penelope would want."
Looking back up I nod, biting my lip as I think about the funeral more. I can hear Lily searching in her purse and grabbing something out of it. Looking back at her she's holding her phone out to me. I must have looked clueless because Lily started to explain why.
"I figured even if you knew a little more than me, you might still need some help."
I nod, grabbing her phone and entering my digits. I hand it back to her, after filing in my name as well. I nod, reaching my hand out.
"It was a pleasure meeting you, Lily"
She grabs my hand with a firmness that I wasn't prepared for. Turning back around I head towards my kids who are still holding onto their mother. I walk over give them a huge hug and pick them up.

Lily's POV

I walk back from meeting with Don and deciding on what to do. The boys seem distraught with what their father said. They notice my heels turn around and start to run at me. I reach their shoulders in a hug and kiss them on the head. I whisper how everything is gonna be alright. My and Don's family walk out side by side and wave when getting into the car.

Chapter 17

Lily's POV

June 13th

I step out of my car and walk up to the home that my dad is staying at. I can hear my heels clicking on the vinyl floors. I walk to the desk with a woman standing behind it with red hair. I wonder if she knew my sister at all. Walking over I stand facing her back waiting until she notices me. I can see her turn around and jump.
"Oh, my lord, you scared me hon!"
"I'm sorry, I am here to see my father.."
"Of course just give me a minute"
I nod, taking in her voice. It's high-pitched and bubbly.
"What's your father's last name?"
"Kyrin"
"Okay, it's down that hall, take a left and you're fourth door on the..uh..on the left!"
I nod as I start to walk off, I notice how my stride is more feeble now. It's strange to me, I normally walk with such pride. But when you just lost a sister then you lose some of your pride.
Getting to my dad's room, it still smells like he did in his 50s. Like wood and cigarettes. He was sitting on a recliner with a quilt draped over him. I noticed him reading a book, The Diving Bell and The Butterfly. My father told me about this book, it was written by a man with locked-in syndrome. The man wrote this by blinking, I believe 200,000 times. And he died shortly after.
"Dad?"
He hums in acknowledgment at me. I take that as an invitation, a lot of time with my father is guessing what he wants. I sit on his bed, with how laid down the covers are it seems he never sleeps. I sigh as I stare at my hands before looking at him.
"Dad, you need to put the book down for this, okay?"
My dad sighs in disappointment, closing the book and playing on the side tale. He looks at me with boredom in his eyes.

"This is a serious goddamn matter!"

I start to get annoyed with how he's not caring about the situation.

"Jesus you don't have to scream"

I can feel my teeth grind together, and my eye twitches in anger. My patient is wearing thin with him, and I suddenly remember why I kept contact with him low.

"This situation is fucking serious and I would appreciate it if you would listen and not give that look"

My voice grows more and more grim as I get more and more angry.

"I fucking am!"

"Penelope's dead"

I didn't want to break the news that way, but I couldn't.

"What...?"

His face lowered after I said that, and his body slumped down into his seat. I nod, not wanting to say anything beforehand.

"What happened?"

"She hung herself..."

"What...?"

He pauses for a minute, his voice going lower in octave. He stops looking at me and starts to look at the floor. I can hear him gulp.

My father and I never really had a good relationship. Penelope was always a mediator when me and dad were fighting. I was rebellious and didn't like how the kids in the school or their moms would talk about my family. I felt judged and angry, but I sent it in the wrong way. When I started to drink and drive my dad stopped caring. The final straw was me getting my boyfriend. A juvenile, vandal, and druggy. He didn't approve, I didn't care and got kicked out.

"She left us a letter, also a friend, but I thought we should read ours together."

"My nurse told me that I got a letter but to not read it until you came"

My dad gets up, wobbly. I feel my body jerking to help him, but I know that he will just push me away. He walks to a dresser with a mirror on the top. He opens the top drawer and digs through the underwear that's in there. He grabs a letter with 'Dad' scribbled in Penelope's handwriting. He sits back down, grunting as he does.

I grab mine out of my purse and trace over the letter in my name with my eyes. I do it again, imagining when Penelope was writing this, and how she weirdly held the pen.

I look at my dad, and he looks at me as well. I nod, and we begin to open the letters. I take care of the envelope so I can keep it later. The sound of ripping fills the room as Dad opens his haphazardly. Closing my eyes I unfold the letter and open them back up. I read each line, with commentary in my mind.

"Dear Lily, When you get this you will probably already know the news"

'No shit, dummy'

"I just wanted to say, it's not your fault"

'I doubt that...'

"This was a very hard decision, but it's what I need"

'No, it's not, you didn't *need* to do this!'

I can feel my body start to shake from crying. My face frowned and my brows furrowed.

"I can't bear to live in this world anymore, there's too much pain."

'I could've helped with your pain! You could've come to me about your problems!'
My body continues to shake as I get father and father into the letter.
"I love you so much, I am sorry that you will have to bear this burden of my death."
'No you asshole, don't apologize, that makes it worse!'
"The one thing I will ask of you is to take care of Dad, and see him more regularly please, he talks so fondly of you."
'I doubt it, but I will for you'
"Love, Your Clone"
I smile at the end and how she signs off. I look up to my father to see what he's doing. His head is resting on the back of the chair. His eyes are closed. The hand that's holding the letter is slowly slipping. I can also see how his face is scrunched up in sadness. And now all I can wonder is what happened with him?

Tom's POV

(Lily's and Penelope's father)

I stare at my bastard daughter as she tells me that my daughter killed herself. She hung herself. My thoughts drift to an image of Penelope sitting here telling me Lily had died. I know I shouldn't feel this way but, if Lily had died I wouldn't have been as distraught. Maybe every parent does have a parent, and mine, Penelope. Lily's voice seems to drown out in a dull buzz. It feels like in a movie, where a person gets flashbacks to happier times, and I can feel that. All of a sudden I am transported back to when she was a kid.
Getting her first camera
Bike riding
Swimming
Baking
I know I put her in a tough position between me and Lily fighting. I wish I could've taken that back. She did need more attention than she had growing up, and a better support system. What I wouldn't give to go back and reassure her that it wasn't her fault.
The only thing I hear from Lily is the portion about a letter. Then it all makes sense, what my nurse explained to me. I wait for her to finish because I don't need her yelling at me anymore.
Getting the letter almost made me realize the reality of this. How my daughter thought about killing herself for a while. Making this plan and carrying it out. It all seems to hit me like a goddamn truck.
Sitting down I see Lily open her letter and she starts to cry. I now start to open mine, I know I'll keep the letter but I don't want the envelope. I can already see her handwriting when I open the letter. Looking at the handwriting reminds me of a letter given to me on fathers day back when she was a kid.
Finally, seeing what the letter is, it's very short.
"Dear Dad,

My life is complete and I love you, take care
-Penelope"
That's all it says.
Some of me wish that it was longer, but others are happy with this. Me and Penelope's relationship was always based on comfortable silence. There was not much talking between us, so it is understandable as to why she wrote it like this. I don't understand why she would do this but I guess I won't ever. I look at Lily, I don't know what I was expecting with her, but seeing her crying was not expected. Since me and her haven't ever been close I don't know what to do in this situation. Deciding that this was my only chance to reconcile with my daughter I got up and moved over to her. She didn't notice me on the bed until I touched her shoulder. I flinched a little before looking at me for a minute. I thought she was gonna scream and hit me, and to be honest I wouldn't blame her. But to my surprise, she hugged me with force. Something I wasn't expecting. In shock for a minute I don't do anything until she shakes with another cry. I hug her back with force and start to cry myself. All I can do is cry, not speak or anything, just tears.
The nurse comes in a little later after we have calmed down and Lily gets up to leave. That's when I heard something that I had been waiting to hear from her...
"I love you dad"
It makes my heart throb with happiness.

Chapter 18

Don's POV
June 13th

Getting back home, I send the kid with their mother. My wife understands that I'll need some alone time right now.

Getting upstairs I loosen my tie and sit on my side of the bed. I take the letter out of my breast pocket. Staring at the writing I flip it over and back over again. I don't understand why I am doing this. Maybe I hope it will change back to the bill that I have to pay and not a suicide note from my friend.

Getting a hold of myself I open the letter and unfold it. I guess what the letter might say but I am at a loss. Never in a million did I think I would be in this position, but no one ever does. Sucking up the courage I read the letter entirely.

"Dear Don,

This was a personal decision that held a lot of thought. Nonetheless, I want to thank you for being my friend. I would be in a much darker place if I didn't have you and your family by my side. I am sorry that I am leaving you, but I hope you hold me dear along with the memories that you have with me.

Love, Penelope"

Once reading I start to beat myself up. I knew that she wasn't happy but I couldn't do anything about it. What kind of friend am I? I could've helped her but I didn't and now she's dead. I didn't realize I had been crying until tear droplets appeared on the letter. I drop the letter entirely and start bawling. I can hear the door open but I don't right now.

"Dad? What's wrong…?"

It's my daughter, I try to explain but all that happens is me blubbering. I cover my face and start to cry more and more. The floor creaks as she moves across the room. The bed barely dips as she sits next to me. She holds onto my arm, wrapping her little arms around my bicep. I reach over with my other hand and cup the back of her head. I press her face next to mine and kiss her. She looks up at me and smiles at me. Again I try to do something but all it ends with is more tears.

I can hear the door open even more. The sound of tennis shoes and heels move across the floor to me and my daughter. It's my wife and son. My son jumps up on the bed on my other side and hugs me. I remove my hand from my daughter's hand and my face. I wrap them around my children and hold them close. My wife holds onto my face and kisses me. I can hear her only a little whispering "It's okay" and "It'll be okay"

We keep holding each other for a while before I go and wipe my face. Thanking them for the help I suggest moving downstairs and looking through some of the stuff she left for us. The kids are excited and rush downstairs while I stay with my wife for a minute.

"Are you gonna be okay, hon?"

"Yeah..I'll be okay"

"Are you sure?"

"Yeah, I am sure, thanks"

I lean over and kiss her, walking downstairs together. The kids are already sitting on the couch with their boxes in hand. The lawyer put Penelope's stuff in boxes for us, each with our name on it.

My son decided to open his first one when we got down the stairs. The box is ripped open to review a collection of acrylic paints, canvas, and watercolor with paint brushes for each. My son's face lights up with excitement about this. One time when we invited Penelope over, she spent 3 hours drawing with my son. It was adorable. That's how she was made into the perfect babysitter. My daughter is next to open up her gifts. It's a collection of books, she is 3 grades higher than her reading level should be. She always wanted more complicated books, but we didn't know what to get her until Penelope. Penelope showed up to her birthday party with a 300-page novel made for kids and my daughter fell in love. She hugged Penelope so tightly that Penelope looked to us for help. So the fact that Penelope held onto all these books for my daughter means a lot. My daughter squeals and hugs the book on the top close to her chest. She looks at us and smiles brightly. I turn to my wife and she starts to open hers with more class than the kids. She reaches in and pulls out a jewelry display bust. As Well as a homemade bracelet dish and an earring holder. My wife gaps in awe at the beauty of the jewelry and touches the jewels. I remember Penelope talking about her father's gifts always being some form of jewelry. I can also remember my wife constantly complimenting Penelope on the jewelry. My wife's mouth is still in shock when she turns to me and smiles in disbelief. She looks back down at the jewelry and smiles greatly at it.
Before I know it all of my family is looking at me. I look around the room to them and then down to the box. Opening the box feels like hours and finally, when I open it, I am at a loss. Looking into the box I see an old Polaroid camera. From the mid-2000s probably. It's pastel pink and full of stickers. I am guessing that she didn't use it for a while until right before her passing. I assume so because the carterged in the back is only missing 2 and it was manufactured in 2018. I look back down into the box to find a stack of Polaroids sitting there. Getting out the polaroids I can see the one on top is a picture of me and her. The funny thing is I don't remember the picture being taken. Looking more closely at the background I can see a ton of beer cans, so it makes sense.
"Why'd she give you that dad?"
I can hear my daughter ask from what feels like miles away.
"Well…Penelope told me a story about the happiest she had ever been. Her 13th birthday, the day after it. Her dad came home late with a cardboard box. The box was falling apart at the seams, with scotch tape on the sides. It was a struggle to open it, but inside was this."
I hold up the camera like a piece of treasure. The kids gasp in awe like it's interesting. The story's not, but all you have to do is play it up with drama and the kids will love it!
"She loved it, she held onto it and brought it everywhere with her. She took pictures of everything. Later when we were hanging out she brought it with her. We took a picture, and I had told her that I wanted something like that when I was younger-"
"In the 1800s?"
That has been my favorite joke for a while now, especially with me. I glance at my wife, only to see her giving my son a hard glare. She glanced back at me, almost asking me for an answer or response. I give her a shrug before getting back to the story.

"Grandma never got me a Polaroid when I asked for one, so when I saw she had one I was ecstatic! I turned back into a kid, and she…she made a joke- a joke about when she's..um..dead…I could have it"
I can feel my smile fall off my face as I keep going with the story. I start to blink more and more thinking of that night. My face races up to face the ceiling as I start to blink even more. I let out a sigh and continued.
"She told me that this would be her gift to me, an old, decrypted version."
I scuff at the memory, and how stupid it seemed at the time but how real it felt now. My bottom lip quivers and I smile again.
"She was a good friend"
I look down at my shoes and I wipe my eyes with a palm as I look over at my kids.
"I am happy you knew her before she passed…"
My wife holds onto the jewelry and leans into me. My head turns and my eyes are focused on a corner in our living room. I kiss her and stay there for a good minute. Turning back around, I grab the Polaroid camera and move to have it point at my wife and me.
Flash
I stand up and walk over to where the kids are getting down on a knee. I hold onto the camera and take another picture.
Flash
Walking over to the kids I sit down again and motion for my wife. She follows over with a smile on her face. She sits next to me, kissing me. I can feel the stickiness of her lip gloss but I don't care. I turn my head a little to show off the shining aspect of it and click the button.
Flash
Flash
Taking back the camera closer to me I take the Polaroid into my hand. I don't shake it because Penelope told me you shouldn't. The family sits around just waiting for it to develop. Once we can all see it, it looks heavenly. The shining of the gloss sparkles and bounces off of my daughter and wife's jewelry. The kids are smiling so big, it looks like it hurts. Cute.
Not every part of this has to be hurt.

-Part 3-

Chapter 19

Lily's POV

June 20th

After a lot of work, we finally got a funeral ready for Penelope. I had worked tirelessly for this to work. To get all the right things, flowers, caskets, pictures, and memorials.
Walking around the church I double-check to make sure everything is in place.
Sighing I move to the back of the church to a closed-off room.
That's where Penelope is.
When I decided that I wanted to have an open casket, we decided to keep it away for the bruising on her neck. That was really what Don decided, thinking that it wouldn't be the best for kids to see a dead body with rope marks on their necks. I decided we would have some of the old Polaroid pictures hanging up as well as some more professional photos. We had her favorite flowers out and present on the table; marigolds. As well as some painting prints that she loved very much. Such as Andy Warhol's Campbell Soup painting.

Walking around there aren't many people but generally enough, about 70. I excuse myself from my husband and dart off to the back room. I close the door and turn around.

There she lies.

Penelope.

Whiter than normal, her veins are more noticeable than before and the obvious rope bruises on her neck. It pains me just to look at her. I crane my neck to the side take a tissue and dap my tears. I walk over and stare at her, she was so pretty when she was alive. Reaching out my hand, I grab onto hers and hold tightly. Maybe I thought that if I hoped enough she would come back to me. I can feel my knees feel weak and I fall. My arms are still on the casket and I hid my face in them. I shake and cry, not caring about my makeup anymore. I whisper about why she left me and let out little wipers in between.

"Sissy…"

The weak sound I hear doesn't even sound like my voice. It sounds feeble. Landing back onto my haunches I slam my hand onto the ground. Trying to let out a scream, but nothing comes out, only a moan of pain. My breathing even sounds like I am in pain. My head rises to stare at the dim lighting of the room. My eyes burn when I don't blink. I can feel the wetness of my tears on my cheeks. My chest feels like it's trying to crush my lungs. It pains me so badly. I can hear a knock at the door and see the shadow of the person entering. My husband wraps his arms around me and picks me up. He drags me out of the room as I continue to cry. I can see the secondhand embarrassment on people's faces but I don't care. My husband continues to carry me out and sit me on a bench. He hands me a tissue and I try to wipe my nose but I am crying so much. Seeing my husband walk around in front of me through blurry eyes is embarrassing. I stopped screaming or whimpering, whatever, and have just been sitting crying. I stare at the ground and all I can think of is;

"Why did she make this so fucking hard on me"

POV TOM

I step into the church where they are holding my 27-year-old daughter's funeral. What the fuck is happening right now.

My finger reaches up to my neck and pulls at the collar. I don't think I've worn a suit in nearly 30 years. Walking around I don't recognize half the people here. Only now am I realizing how out of touch I was with my daughter. Even with our comfort in silence, I never cared to ask about her. I am a horrible dad.

Walking around I try not to seem awkward and move to the snack table. It's full of crap, finger sandwiches, and charcuterie boards. I poke around with a toothpick and decide to just eat a grape. Hearing some ruckus behind me I turn to see Lily being dragged out by her husband. She was screaming and crying about Penelope I assume. Looking to where she was running from it has a sign near it. It reads, 'Open casket' looking back through the window to Lily. She's sitting on a bench, hunched over with what looks like pain. Sighing I move myself over to the room. Getting inside the room, I can see some teardrops on the casket. Going over to the casket, I see Penelope. It takes me a minute to stop staring at her face and move down to the rope ark that's around her neck. It's purple and blue, disgusting looking. Penelope looks peaceful, and quiet where she finds herself.
She looks almost happy.
Grabbing her hand there is still some warmth from Lily grabbing it. I look down at my hand and see the shimmer on my finger. It's my old wedding ring. I never took it off. Looking back at Penelope's face, I start to think.
Would I be okay with this ring being buried in the ground?
If it was with Penelope then yes I would be okay with it. I would be more than okay with it.
Letting go of her hand I took a look at mine by itself. Taking the ring off I take a look at it more closely. It's silver and it has a floral design. When Penelope was a kid she would take it off and wear it. Or she would just admire it on my finger. I smile and slide it on her hand, it doesn't fit her ring finger but it does fit her middle finger. Sliding it on I bring her hand to my mouth. I kiss the ring and place her hand back gently.
I smile and walk out of the room. Closing the door, I look down at my ring finger which now has a pale line across my tan skin. Closing my eyes and resting my head against the door I take a breath and leave.

POV DON

Walking into the church was weird, some people I recognized. Like Barbra from behind the desk. And some people I don't know.
I send my kids and my wife to the snack table as I leave to find Penelope's casket. Walking around the church I spot things that I suggested and things Lily did for this. Walking around even more I see the room where Penelope is. Walking in I close the door behind me. Walking over I look at Penelope's face. Seeing her like this almost feels like a different person. Looking around at the casket and her I notice something. It's a silver ring on her middle finger. I touch it for a second before removing it. I look around it before checking the insides. There's an inscription, that says,
"For our daughters"
I assume this is a wedding ring from her father. It's pretty, I slip it back on her finger.

Looking back up to her face I notice that they put some makeup on her. I told them not to, Penelope was never one to care what she looked like so I don't why they did this. Getting out a makeup wipe that I hold for my wife, I start to wipe the makeup away. Her true beauty is coming through. Her freckles and beauty mark, there they are. Smiling, I step back and grab something out of my front pocket.
Taking two pictures of my family with the Polaroid was planned for this. Taking out the second one of my family I place it on Penelope's sternum. It just feels right to have this with her.
I stand at the door and look over her one more time before leaving. Getting out of the room, my kids come up with another plate of food. Taking it from them I mess with their hair and walk over to a pew. Watching my kids follow me with their mother fills my heart with love. Sitting here there is no sadness, it's not mourning Penelope's death, it's celebrating her life. Regardless of what happens my kids are going to learn about their aunt.
How good of a person she was
How kind
How creative
How funny
How she was an amazing friend
Looking back up at the stained glass I stare at the colors. Penelope loved stained glass, and how pretty it was. I smile and eat a grape, looking back down at my kids I smile and hold onto them.

Penelope will forever live on in our memory.

A Novel
By: Matilda Reese

www.ingramcontent.com/pod-product-compliance
Lightning Source LLC
Chambersburg PA
CBHW051711250726
48653CB00007B/2970